CHILBLAINS

Guidelines for Preventing Chilblains: Ensuring Warmth and Protection for the Extremities

CARL JUAN

Table of Contents

Introductory

Chilblains, also known as pernio, are caused by the inflammation of small blood vessels in the skin and are a common reaction to extreme cold. Chilblains, an injury caused by exposure to cold, are more prevalent in northern latitudes.

- Chilblains are characterized by patches of red, itchy, swollen, and painful skin, most frequently on the fingers, toes, ears, and nose. Discoloration, blistering, and even ulceration of the skin are possible side effects. Cold temperatures followed by rapid warming can cause a localized inflammatory response in the skin, resulting in chilblains.

• Keeping the extremities warm, avoiding sudden temperature fluctuations, and keeping the blood flowing well are common preventative measures against chilblains. In severe or persistent occurrences, it's recommended to seek medical assistance, as complications can arise, such as infection or tissue damage. Chilblains are a mild form of cold injury, but frostbite, in which the skin and underlying tissues are damaged, is much more serious.

CHAPTER ONE
Factors and Causes

Chilblains are generally linked to being in cold and moist environments, while the specific etiology is unclear. Blood vessels close to the skin's surface constrict (narrow) when the skin cools down, which helps the body retain heat. When these narrowed blood vessels don't respond quickly to rewarming, an aberrant response of the blood vessels and surrounding tissues can occur, and chilblains can develop. Inflammation and damage to localized tiny blood vessels are possible outcomes.

• Chilblains are most common in cold weather, especially when the temperature is hovering around or below freezing. An increase in risk is associated with sudden exposure to cold weather, such as going outside without enough clothes.

• High humidity and moist circumstances might promote the growth of chilblains. The skin's protective barrier may be compromised by excessive moisture.

• Chilblains are more common in those who have impaired circulation, which can be caused by illnesses like Raynaud's disease or diabetes. Poor circulation might hinder the body's ability to adjust to sudden temperature shifts.

• There may be a genetic propensity for chilblains in some people. If chilblains run in your family, you may be at a higher risk.

• Chilblains occur more frequently in females than males.

• **Clothing**: Chilblains are more likely to occur in people who wear clothes that are too tight or too restricting and don't give enough insulation and protection from the cold.

• **Cigarette smoking:** Cigarette smoking has been shown to reduce blood flow and increase the risk of developing chilblains.

• If you've suffered from chilblains before, you might be more prone to getting them again.

Keep in mind that chilblains are only transitory and will go away on their own after a few weeks of keeping the affected regions warm and dry. However, if your chilblains are really severe or you have them frequently, you should see a doctor to rule out more serious problems. Avoiding chilblains can be done by taking precautions including staying warm, dressing appropriately, and keeping the skin away from wet and chilly environments.

Acute Symptoms

Chilblains are a skin condition that are more common in colder climates. Chilblains typically manifest themselves by the following:

1. One of the first symptoms of chilblains is a crimson or bluish-red appearance of the affected skin.

2. Extreme itching is a common symptom of chilblains. The itching can range from minor to severe and be very annoying.

3. Swelling: The skin in the affected area may become swollen or puffy. Oftentimes, a warm or burning sensation will accompany this swelling.

4. Chilblains can cause a lot of discomfort. Pain is often characterized as sensitive or scorching and can be exacerbated by heat.

5. Chilblains can cause tiny blisters on the skin in some people. In severe situations, the blisters may burst, exposing the underlying skin and causing peeling or ulceration.

6. Discoloration of the Skin: Chilblains can cause skin to become mottled, darker, or purple in the affected area.

7. Skin Ulcers and Sores might form in Severe Cases or when Chilblains Persist. These wounds, being open, are susceptible to infection.

8. Skin in the affected area may become sensitive, making it painful or uncomfortable to apply pressure.

Chilblains are a form of frostbite that affect the skin of the fingers, toes, ears, and nose. In most cases, the symptoms appear anywhere from a few hours to a few days after being exposed to cold and damp weather. While chilblains can be irritating, they are generally not a significant medical problem and often resolve on their own within a few weeks after the affected areas are routinely kept warm and dry. Seek medical assistance if your symptoms worsen or continue, especially if you develop open sores, as these are more likely to lead to complications like infection.

CHAPTER TWO
Safety and Security Measures

Protecting your skin from cold and moist environments is the most important thing you can do to avoid getting chilblains. Here are some ways to lessen your chances of getting chilblains:

1. Layer up for warmth and make sure your fingers and toes are protected from the cold by wearing socks and gloves or shoes. Put on some warm gloves, some thick socks, and some waterproof boots.

2. Chilblains are more likely to develop if there is any moisture on the skin. Keep your clothes and shoes dry, and if you can, wear waterproof ones.

3. Try not to experience sudden shifts in temperature and give your body time to adjust to the cold. Chilblains are more likely to occur when the skin is rapidly warmed after being exposed to cold or when the skin is cold to begin with.

4. Proper Footwear: Insulated and waterproof footwear can help protect your feet from cold and wetness. It's important to wear properly sized shoes or boots to avoid discomfort.

5. Instead of immediately applying heat to cold skin, it's best to let your body warm up gradually after coming in from the cold.

6. Avoid or at least cut down on smoking, as this habit might impede blood flow and leave you more vulnerable to chilblains.

7. Regular exercise can assist improve circulation, which in turn reduces the likelihood of developing chilblains.

8. Reduce Your Caffeine And Alcohol Intake Both substances can narrow blood arteries, which can lead to poor blood flow. It could be advantageous to reduce consumption.

9. Keep Rooms Warm: Maintain a warm interior atmosphere during cold weather. Don't let the temperature inside your home drop too low before turning on the heaters or the furnace.

10. Apply Moisturizers: Dry, cracked skin is more prone to chilblains, therefore it's important to keep your skin hydrated.

11. Keep in mind that some drugs can have an effect on blood flow. If you are concerned that any of the medications you are currently taking may increase your risk of chilblains, you should speak with your doctor.

12. Consult your doctor often if you have a condition that affects your circulation, such as Raynaud's syndrome or diabetes.

Keep in mind that while these methods might greatly lessen the likelihood of contracting chilblains, they may not provide complete protection, particularly in extremely cold and moist climates. Chilblains can cause serious problems if not treated quickly. Seek professional medical advice if your symptoms worsen or continue, especially if you have any reason to suspect infection.

Care and Handling

Chilblains are a common skin condition that can be treated and managed such that symptoms are reduced, healing is accelerated, and complications are avoided.

• The initial step is to apply gentle heat to the injured areas. If you want to keep from getting burned, stay away from heaters and radiators. Instead, try relocating to a warmer location or soaking the affected limbs in warm (not hot) water.

• Reduce swelling and increase blood flow by propping up the affected limbs by elevating them. If your toes are hurting, for instance, you should elevate them.

• After gently warming the damaged regions, you should pat them dry and cover them so they don't get any colder or wetter. Put on some warm, dry clothes and shoes.

• OTC creams and ointments, such as corticosteroid creams, can be used to the affected area to provide temporary relief from itching and irritation. Follow the instructions on the product's label and visit a healthcare provider if you're unsure.

• Resist the impulse to scratch the affected regions; doing so may make your condition worse and even cause permanent skin damage or infection.

• Over-the-counter pain medicines, such as ibuprofen or acetaminophen, may provide some relief from discomfort and suffering. Always go by the suggested dosages.

• To avoid further skin dryness and cracking, moisturize the afflicted areas with a lotion or cream.

• Trim and file your nails regularly to avoid touching the sore skin and spreading infection.

• Chilblains should be evaluated and treated by a medical professional if the symptoms are severe, if open sores or other evidence of infection appear, or if the condition does not improve with self-care. If necessary, they can prescribe medication or suggest other advanced treatments.

• Make sure you don't get chilblains again by following the steps in the "Prevention and Risk Reduction" section once you've recovered from them. Some of these are maintaining body heat, preventing moisture loss, and covering exposed skin to prevent frostbite.

Chilblains, when treated properly, usually go away on their own within a few weeks. However, there is considerable variation in the severity of the illness, and problems may arise if it is not treated. If your symptoms are severe or aren't getting better, you should see a doctor. Chilblain risk can also be reduced in those who have underlying medical problems that impact circulation, such as Raynaud's disease, but only if they work with their doctors to do so.

CHAPTER THREE
Therapeutic Procedures

Self-care and home treatments, such as those already suggested, are usually sufficient for treating chilblains. However, medical measures may be required when chilblains are severe, chronic, or complicated. Examples of such measures could be:

• If the chilblains are exceptionally painful or severe, a doctor may prescribe medicine to assist alleviate symptoms and reduce inflammation. Sometimes doctors will recommend a course of oral or topical corticosteroids.

- Prescription-strength topical creams or ointments may be prescribed for symptom alleviation and inflammation reduction, in addition to over-the-counter choices.

- **Wound Care:** If chilblains have grown into open sores or ulcers, wound care may be needed. To avoid infection, it may be necessary to clean the wounds, apply antibacterial creams, and cover them with sterile coverings.

- **Antibiotics:** develop the event that an infection sets develop from chilblains, antibiotics may be prescribed.

- **Vasodilators**: Vasodilator drugs that enlarge blood arteries may be considered for those with severe or recurrent chilblains, particularly if they are connected with disorders like Raynaud's illness.

- Chilblains can sometimes be treated with cryotherapy (cold therapy) administered by medical specialists. Applying ice to the injured area in a regulated manner can help alleviate inflammation and speed recovery.

- In extreme cases of chilblains, a dermatologist may offer phototherapy (treatment with certain wavelengths of light) to alleviate symptoms and boost blood flow to the affected areas.

It's crucial to remember that medical procedures are normally reserved for cases when chilblains are very severe, painful, or difficult, as most chilblains will cure with basic self-care and preventative measures. If you have chilblains and are worried about the severity of your symptoms or the risk of consequences, you should see a doctor to get an accurate diagnosis and advice on how to treat the condition.

Handling Difficulties

Although chilblains are typically harmless, they can occasionally cause more serious issues. The health and well-being of the affected person depends on effective management of these problems. Common chilblain complications and their treatments are outlined below.

1. Infection: Chilblains can produce open sores or ulcers, which can get infected. Seek immediate medical assistance if you have any of the following symptoms of infection: increasing redness, warmth, swelling, discharge, or worsening discomfort. Antibiotics are a possible course of treatment suggested by your doctor.

2. Skin ulcers are a possible complication of severe chilblains. It is essential to clean and dress these ulcers with sterile materials. Follow your doctor's instructions for wound care, including changing the dressings on a regular basis. It's crucial to keep the area clean and prevent any additional damage.

3. Chilblains can cause scarring if they are scratched or rubbed, so take care to avoid doing either. Proper wound care and protection against infection can lessen the likelihood of scarring. Scars may diminish with time, but if you're self-conscious about how they look, a dermatologist can help.

4. Tissue damage can occur in extreme and prolonged cases of chilblains. In severe circumstances, this can lead to skin necrosis (the death of skin tissue). Wound care, and in rare situations referral to a specialist for additional evaluation and possible therapies, may be part of the management of tissue damage.

5. It is important to work closely with your healthcare professional to manage the underlying illness if you are suffering recurring chilblains or if they are related with other health concerns like Raynaud's disease. Medication or behavioral changes may be suggested to enhance circulation and lessen the likelihood of chilblains.

6. Preventing chilblains is the most effective method for dealing with any issues that may arise. Maintaining a warm and dry environment and wrapping your extremities in protective clothing can help prevent chilblains and its complications.

Chilblains and their complications, whether they are severe or continue for an extended period of time, require quick medical intervention. A medical professional is in the best position to diagnose your problem, suggest therapies, and advise you on wound care and prevention. Additionally, for those with underlying health issues that predispose them to chilblains, continual therapy and surveillance are crucial to limit the risk of complications.

CHAPTER FOUR
Managing Recurrent Chilblains

Recurrent or persistent chilblains are known as chronic chilblains, and they can be difficult to manage. Here are some methods for enhancing your quality of life while efficiently managing your condition:

1. If your chilblains persist for an extended period of time, you should see a doctor, preferably a dermatologist or rheumatologist. They will be able to diagnose your illness, pin down its origins and choose the best course of treatment for you.

2. Medication: Depending on the reason of your chronic chilblains, your doctor may give vasodilators (drugs that dilate blood vessels) or anti-inflammatory treatments to help alleviate your symptoms.

3. Lifestyle Modifications: Make lifestyle adjustments to lower your risk of chilblains. This may involve avoiding cold or wet conditions or extreme temperatures. Giving up nicotine and cutting back on stimulants like caffeine and alcohol can also be beneficial.

4. Warm Clothing: Invest in high-quality, warm clothing and accessories, such as insulated gloves, socks, and footwear. Wrap up warmly in many thin layers of clothing.

5.Be sure your shoes are warm, waterproof, and a suitable fit for the chilly weather ahead. To enhance blood flow to the feet, orthotic insoles may be suggested.

6. Transitioning from a chilly to a warm environment requires a measured approach. Give your skin and limbs a chance to acclimate to the cold before venturing out.

7. Maintaining clean, dry, and moisturized feet is an important part of healthy foot care. Do not

venture out into the cold with bare feet.

8. Warm water soaks or electric blankets are great ways to gradually warming up chilly limbs. Stay away from anything that could possibly burn you.

9. Maintain regular check-ups with your doctor if you have a preexisting condition like Raynaud's, diabetes, or a circulatory disorder, and do as they advise for treatment.

10. Chilblains can be made worse by stress, so learning to deal with that is important. Take part in stress-reduction activities like yoga, meditation, or relaxation techniques to better handle your condition.

11. Determine what makes your chilblains worse, and try to steer clear of those things. This may include certain meals, environmental circumstances, or activities that exacerbate your symptoms.

12. Join a support group or online community for those who suffer from chilblains or a similar condition. The advice and comfort of those who have been through similar situations is invaluable.

13. Nutrition & Diet: Eat a healthy, well-balanced diet that helps keep your blood flowing smoothly. If you have any questions or concerns about your nutrition, talk to your doctor or a dietitian.

If you suffer from chronic chilblains, you and your doctor should work together to develop a treatment plan that best suits your situation. Keep in mind that although dealing with persistent chilblains can be upsetting, many people are able to find efficient ways to manage their disease and limit the burden on their everyday lives.

The Influence of the Season on Chilblains

Chilblains are more frequently linked with cold temperatures, but they can be an issue during seasonal changes especially in milder areas. Chilblains are seasonal, so keep these things in mind:

1. Chilblains occur most frequently during the winter months because to the cold and moist conditions. To avoid getting chilblains this winter, it's important to bundle up, wear clothing designed for the cold, and keep your fingers and toes dry and warm.

2. When temperatures rise and fall rapidly, as they do in autumn and spring, chilblains are a common symptom. Keep an eye on the thermometer and work to gradually accustom your body to the different temperatures so that you don't get too chilled all at once. Keep dry, as wetness can make chilblains worse.

3. Summer: The warmer temperatures mean fewer cases of chilblains. Chilblains are typically associated with the winter season, but in some milder and more humid places, they can occur in the summer if the temperature abruptly turns chilly. When temperatures drop suddenly, it's crucial to be prepared with warm clothing and safety measures.

4. If your travels take you to areas with wildly different climates, pack accordingly. Bring along warm garments and adjust your attire accordingly for the predicted weather.

5. Indoor Heating: Be cautious with indoor heating during colder seasons. Chilblains may be particularly susceptible to temperature changes if they are exposed to overly warm and dry circumstances, as can occur in overheated interior areas. Make sure the temperature inside stays nice and steady.

6. During the winter months, greater care must be used when engaging in outdoor sports or activities. Wear warm, water-resistant clothing and footwear that is suited for outdoor exercise in the cold.

7. Children and Vulnerable Individuals: Children and individuals with specific medical problems, such as diabetes or Raynaud's illness, may be more prone to chilblains. It's crucial that they be kept warm and dry and that they have the right clothing for the weather.

8. Maintaining Preventative Measures: Preventative measures against chilblains should be maintained year-round. Some of these measures include not becoming too chilly, not getting too wet, dressing in layers, and covering exposed skin.

Keep in mind that chilblains can happen at any time of year, but are especially common in cold, damp climates. It's vital to remain aware, practice proper self-care, and take actions to prevent chilblains year-round, especially if you have a history of the condition or are at higher risk. If you get chilblains, you should treat them right away so that the pain goes away and any problems are avoided.

CHAPTER FIVE

Contrasting Chilblains with Other Cold-Related Illnesses

Chilblains are a sort of cold-associated skin disorder, but there are a number of others that share some of the same symptoms or are somehow related to the cold. Here are some similarities and differences between chilblains and other cold-related illnesses:

1. Frostbite:

Chilblains: These painful, red, itchy, swollen patches of skin are the result of an inappropriate skin response to cold. Chilblains are a skin condition that commonly manifest on the hands, feet, ears, and nose.

Extreme cold can cause frostbite, a condition in which the skin and its underlying tissues freeze and die. The affected area may freeze, leading to numbness, discolouration, and damage that may be so severe that it causes tissue death.

2. Its called Raynaud's phenomenon or Raynaud's disease.

• Chilblains: Raynaud's illness, in which the fingers and toes change color intermittently in response to cold or stress, is sometimes linked to chilblains. Chilblains are a potential side effect of Raynaud's illness.

• Color changes, tingling, and discomfort in the fingers and toes are all symptoms of Raynaud's illness, a disorder in which the tiny blood capillaries in these extremities constrict in response to cold or stress. Chilblains are a possible side effect of Raynaud's, but they are different from the disease itself.

3. Immersion Foot or Trench Foot:

- Chilblains are an abnormal reaction of the skin to cold and moist environments. They have nothing to do with being submerged in cold water for a long time.

When the feet are subjected to cold, wet, and filthy circumstances for an extended period of time, a condition known as trench foot can develop. Unlike chilblains, it can cause swelling, blisters, and numbness due to tissue injury.

4. Icy Urticaria:

• Inflammation and redness of the skin, known as chilblains, are common symptoms of prolonged exposure to cold and moist conditions.

When exposed to cold temperatures, such as those found in cold air or water, some people develop a skin condition known as cold urticaria, characterized by hives, itching, and redness. It's a physical urticaria, but it doesn't always look like chilblains.

Differentiating between these disorders is essential due to the fact that their root causes, symptoms, and treatments may differ. In the event that you have skin issues due to the cold or are unsure of your condition, it is best to see a doctor. Accurate diagnosis is vital for identifying the right management and treatment for your unique ailment.

Conclusion

chilblains are a skin ailment caused by prolonged exposure to cold and damp weather. They often result in red, itchy, swollen, and painful regions on the skin, most commonly affecting the extremities like fingers, toes, ears, or nose. Although chilblains are annoying, they are usually not life-threatening and will go away after a few weeks of treatment.

- Preventing chilblains entails staying warm, keeping dry, and protecting your skin from the cold. Self-care measures for chilblains include warming the affected regions, keeping them dry, and applying over-the-counter treatments. Medication and medical intervention may be required if symptoms are particularly severe or persistent.

• Recurrent or persistent chilblains, known as chronic chilblains, may call for on-going treatment and investigation into any underlying health issues. You and your doctor should collaborate together to develop a treatment strategy that is just right for you.

Keep in mind that the key to successful chilblain management is a prompt and correct diagnosis. You

should see a doctor if your
symptoms are worrying you or if
they aren't getting better despite
treatment.

THE END